Hèla Ben Jmaà
Fatma Boudaya

# Aorto-femoral bypass surgery

Hèla Ben Jmaà
Fatma Boudaya

# Aorto-femoral bypass surgery

## Abdominal aorta bypass grafts

ScienciaScripts

**Imprint**

Any brand names and product names mentioned in this book are subject to trademark, brand or patent protection and are trademarks or registered trademarks of their respective holders. The use of brand names, product names, common names, trade names, product descriptions etc. even without a particular marking in this work is in no way to be construed to mean that such names may be regarded as unrestricted in respect of trademark and brand protection legislation and could thus be used by anyone.

Cover image: www.ingimage.com

This book is a translation from the original published under ISBN 978-620-6-72063-8.

Publisher:
Sciencia Scripts
is a trademark of
Dodo Books Indian Ocean Ltd. and OmniScriptum S.R.L publishing group

120 High Road, East Finchley, London, N2 9ED, United Kingdom
Str. Armeneasca 28/1, office 1, Chisinau MD-2012, Republic of Moldova, Europe
Printed at: see last page
**ISBN: 978-620-8-04219-6**

# *AORTO-FEMORAL BYPASS SURGERY*

# I- INTRODUCTION

Atherosclerotic occlusive disease of the aortic junction and iliac axes is the preferred site for atherosclerotic disease, which is a general disease that can affect all medium- and large-calibre arteries [1].

The management of these patients has benefited from advances in diagnostic imaging based on ultrasound, CT and angiographic scans. The treatment options for aorto-iliac occlusive disease are endovascular treatment and surgical treatment, both of which have undergone considerable development, aided by increasingly sophisticated imaging techniques.Endovascular treatment is indicated mainly for focal lesions of moderate length, whereas surgery is indicated for patients with long, multiple lesions. This surgery is associated with a significant morbidity and mortality rate, dominated by cardiac and digestive complications.

# II- EPIDEMIOLOGY

## 1- Frequency :

It is a common pathology throughout the world, particularly in older people with cardiovascular risk factors. Numerous studies have been carried out over the last 20 years to define the prevalence of this disease, which is estimated at 1% before the age of 50, and over 7% after the age of 60 [2].

In the German epidemiological study on Ankle Brachial Index, one in five patients was considered to have arterial disease over the age of 65 [3].

In Africa, rapid and uncontrolled urbanisation and major lifestyle changes are at the root of the rising prevalence of diabetes, obesity and arterial hypertension, which are the main risk factors for lower limb arterial disease [4].

## 2- Age :

It is well established that cardiovascular risk increases with age. According to the Criqui study [5], 2.5% of patients aged under 60, 8.3% of patients aged between 60 and 69, and 18.8% of patients aged over 70 had arterial disease. The Boccalon study [6] in France showed a prevalence of the disease of 8% in patients aged under 50, compared with 13.3% in subjects aged over 80. The probability of arteritis, all other factors being equal, increased by 23% for each 10-year age bracket. The average age of the patient at the time of diagnosis is around 50.

## 3- Gender :

Obliterative arteriopathy of the lower limbs is more common in men than in women during the reproductive period, with a sex ratio varying from 1 to 8 [7]. After the menopause, the level of risk in women gradually approaches that in men.The Créqui study [5] screened 613 patients in southern California for arterial disease, and found that the sex ratio varied with patient age, but was still predominantly male, with an average of 1.3.

**4- Risk factors :**

There are 6 main risk factors directly involved in the pathogenesis of atherosclerosis: smoking, hypertension, diabetes, dyslipidaemia, heredity and age [8].

There are other factors that increase cardiovascular risk because they favour the major risk factors. These are: obesity, sedentary lifestyle, nutritional factors, psychosocial factors and chronic renal failure [9].

**- Smoking:** Smoking is a key risk factor in aorto-ilio-femoral atherogenesis [10]. It increases cardiovascular morbidity and mortality, which depends on the dose and duration of exposure.

According to the Edinburg Artery Study, a randomised trial involving 1,592 patients aged 55 to 74, the relative risk of developing arterial disease was 3.7 times greater in smokers than in non-smokers [11].

**- Hypertension:** Hypertension is a major cardiovascular risk factor, defined as systolic blood pressure = 140 mm Hg and/or diastolic blood pressure = 90 mm Hg on 2 separate visits. The link between blood pressure and cardiovascular risk is continuous.

The United Kingdom prospective diabetes study (UKPDS) showed that a 10 mm Hg increase in systolic blood pressure was associated with a 25% increase in the risk of stroke [12].

**- Diabetes:** Diabetes mellitus is one of the most common non-communicable diseases in the world today. It is a major cardiovascular risk factor that has become epidemic in several countries [13].

There is a clear association between diabetes and the increased prevalence of obliterative arterial disease of the lower limbs. Diabetic patients are 4 to 6 times more likely to develop peripheral arterial disease than non-diabetics.

In the San Luis Valley Diabetes Study, 13.7% of diabetic patients had arterial disease [14].

The UKPDS showed that a 1% increase in HbA1c was associated with a 28% increase in the risk of developing peripheral arterial disease [12].

- **Dyslipidaemia:** Numerous studies have demonstrated the indisputable role of plasma cholesterol and its fractions in cardiovascular disease caused by atherosclerosis.

The detrimental role of its various fractions depends on whether there is an increase in LDL cholesterol, a decrease in HDL cholesterol and a total cholesterol/HDL cholesterol ratio > 4.5 [15].

The Framingham study showed that the increase in total cholesterol levels increased with the incidence of intermittent claudication [16].

Family history: The Framingham study showed that the occurrence of a cardiovascular death in a parent increased the risk of coronary heart disease in children by 30% [17].

- **Excess weight:** Increased body fat (obesity and overweight) is a public health problem. Excess abdominal fat is also associated with cardiovascular risk.

- **Other risk factors:** a sedentary lifestyle, stress and psycho-social factors, hyper-homocysteinemia, thrombogenic factors such as elevated fibrinogen levels, chronic renal failure....

**5- Associated lesions :**

There is a correlation between AOMI and other locations of atheromatous arterial stenosis, as the risk factors for these pathologies are identical, as is their pathophysiology. According to the REACH study, which is a prospective, observational study conducted over 2 years in 44 countries and including 67888 patients aged over 45 with coronary, cerebral or lower limb vascular disease, a combination of at least 2 vascular pathologies was observed in 15.9% of cases [18].

- **Renal artery stenosis:** the association of an aorto-iliac lesion with stenosis of a renal artery is frequent: association with stenosis $\geq$ 70% of at least one main renal artery occurs in 15 to 30% of cases, and association with bilateral lesions occurs in 5 to 20% of cases [19].

- **Stenosis of the digestive arteries:** this stenosis is often associated with the aorto-iliac occlusive lesion, but is often asymptomatic. It is only revealed postoperatively in the form of intestinal gangrene. In some patients with atherosclerosis of the superior mesenteric artery who undergo aorto-iliac revascularisation, intestinal ischaemia may not occur until months or years later [20].

- **Carotid artery stenosis:** According to J.P. Leschi [21], the following rates can be assumed for the association of OAMI with asymptomatic lesions of the extra-cranial internal carotid artery:

Stenosis = 50% or occlusion: 30 to 36% (compared with 2 to 6% in the general population)

Stenosis = 70%: 8 to 12%.

Occlusion: 5 to 8%.

- **Coronary artery stenosis:** According to L. Chiche [22], the prevalence of coronary insufficiency in candidates for aorto-iliac surgery for arteriopathy of the lower limbs is between 21% and 33%.

# III- CLINICAL STUDY

## 1- Circumstances of discovery :

The diagnosis of OSA can be established by questioning, clinical examination and non-invasive para-clinical tests [23].

Arteriopathy may be completely asymptomatic, discovered during a systematic examination, whether or not it is guided by associated atheromatous pathology.

Asymptomatic AOMI has a haemodynamic definition: an ankle/arm systolic pressure index of less than or equal to 0.9 [24].

In the Rotterdam study, 99.4% of subjects with an SPI equal to or greater than 0.90 had no intermittent claudication, whereas only 6.3% of subjects with an SPI less than 0.90 had claudication [25].

Intermittent claudication is a progressively painful cramp-like discomfort, most often in the calf, which increases with the duration or speed of walking and eventually forces the patient to stop, causing the pain to disappear within a few minutes. The intensity of the pain varies, as does its location: it can also affect the buttocks, thighs or soles of the feet. A reduction in walking perimeter is indicative of worsening ischaemia. Intermittent claudication is the classic clinical symptom, but only affects 10% to 35% of patients with OAMI [26].

The Leriche and Fontaine classification is a clinical classification into 4 stages:

- Stage I: asymptomatic, and on clinical examination: abolition of one or more pulses.

- Stage II: intermittent claudication: cramp-like pain that occurs progressively during walking, in a specific muscle area, most often the calf. This pain increases as the patient continues to walk, and its intensity forces the patient to stop. It disappears in less than 10 minutes after stopping the effort, and reappears when it is resumed, after the same distance.

- Stage III: decubitus pain (permanent ischaemia).

It is a distal pain which starts in the toes, appears after a variable period of decubitus, the shorter the period, the more severe the arterial insufficiency, and is relieved by putting the limb in orthostasis, causing the patient to get up once or several times a night, then forcing him to keep the leg dangling. It is very intense and resistant to painkillers, indicating permanent ischaemia linked to extensive arterial lesions, with a serious prognosis and requiring urgent treatment.

- Stage IV: These may be expressed in a number of ways and be of varying degrees of severity: arterial ulcer, necrosis of the toe or even gangrene.

In critical ischaemia, pain occurs a few hours after decubitus, and is relieved by placing the limb in a horizontal position. This hanging-leg position causes stasis oedema, aggravating the circulatory insufficiency.

Trophic disorders are the result of permanent ischaemia leading to tissue necrosis. These are gangrene or ulcers. Gangrene affects the extremities. It may be spontaneous or caused by trauma. It begins at the pulp of the toes and extends more or less upwards. Necrosis is dry, but may become moist if superinfection occurs.Ischaemic ulcers are often painful and occur on the foot, ankle or leg. They are necrotic, atonic and vary in size.Acute or sub-acute forms are less frequent than chronic forms, and are associated with acute thrombosis of the aorta. Acute occlusion of the sub-renal aorta is due either to an embolus obstructing the entire aortic arch, or to acute thrombosis of pre-existing stenoses. The clinical presentation can be misleading; it is not uncommon for the patient to be referred to neurology for an extensive sensory-motor deficit of the lower limbs, or even to general surgery for a pelvic syndrome.

## 2- Physical examination :

The physical examination must be bilateral and comparative. It is based on :

- Inspection of both lower limbs

- Palpation of peripheral pulses

- Measurement of the systolic pressure index: the SPI is now an integral part of arterial investigation of the lower limbs, and has been incorporated into the definitions of OAMI, which take account of both the clinical and haemodynamic impact of the obliterating atheromatous lesion. It provides information on the quality of blood perfusion to the ankle and assesses the haemodynamic impact of any upstream arterial lesions. Below 0.90, the SPI indicates an OAMI with a sensitivity of 95% and a specificity close to 100% [27]. Above 1.30, it defines media-calcosis of the leg. It is also useful for monitoring the development of arterial disease under treatment.

# IV- ADDITIONAL TESTS

Imaging of the abdominal aorta and the arteries of the lower limbs has evolved considerably in recent years, with the use of computed tomography (CT) and magnetic resonance imaging (MRI). Imaging has made progress in both diagnostic and therapeutic terms, with the advent of endovascular treatments for aorto-iliac occlusive disease.

**1- Arterial Doppler ultrasound :**

It is a non-invasive examination that provides morphological and haemodynamic information, which can be combined to quantify a stenosis and study the downstream arterial bed. It is currently the first-line examination carried out in patients with OAMI. Protocols for performing arterial Doppler ultrasound of the lower limbs vary from one team to another, as do the criteria used to diagnose stenoses.

- Standard two-dimensional mode: used to analyse vascular morphology. The vessel has an anechoic lumen and an echogenic wall, the thickness, regularity and any calcifications of which are assessed in axial or longitudinal section in relation to the vessel axis.

- The pulsed Doppler mode analyses the speed of blood flow: the value of the speeds recorded at the level of a stenosis, upstream and downstream, is a function of the degree of this stenosis.

- Colour Doppler codes the column of blood circulating in the artery according to a colour scale linked to the speed and direction of blood flow. This colour mapping identifies the area of acceleration or turbulence generated by the stenosis.

This is an imaging technique using ultrasound, so it is non-irradiating, non-invasive and can be performed at the patient's bedside. It is an operator-dependent examination. Doppler ultrasound quantification of stenoses and occlusions in AOMI therefore comes up against technical difficulties. The patient's condition is assessed on the basis of the following criteria: diffusion of lesions, calcifications preventing ultrasound penetration, excess weight, digestive interpositions, skin lesions and scars, oedema, limited patient mobility hindering visualisation of arterial axes. It is used to characterise the type of lesion (stenosis or obliteration), its topography and its haemodynamic impact. It can also be used to monitor the progress of treatment.

## 2- Angioscan :

Given the invasive nature of arteriography, angioscanner has become the benchmark examination for making an accurate assessment of the lesions and establishing the therapeutic indication.The principle is to obtain a series of successive millimetre thin sections during venous opacification of vascular structures, and to juxtapose the images in order to reconstruct the vascular anatomy [28].

This can be achieved without difficulty on multi-bar equipment because of the speed of acquisition.It is a rapid and readily available test, very useful in emergencies. Its disadvantages are radiation exposure and the nephrotoxicity of iodinated contrast products. One of the advantages of a CT scan is that it allows us to study not only the arterial lumen, but also to visualise atheromatous plaque within the arterial wall. It can be used to detect calcifications in the aorta and its branches, in particular the renal arteries, visceral arteries and arteries of the lower limbs. It can also be used to study the state of collateral circulation.

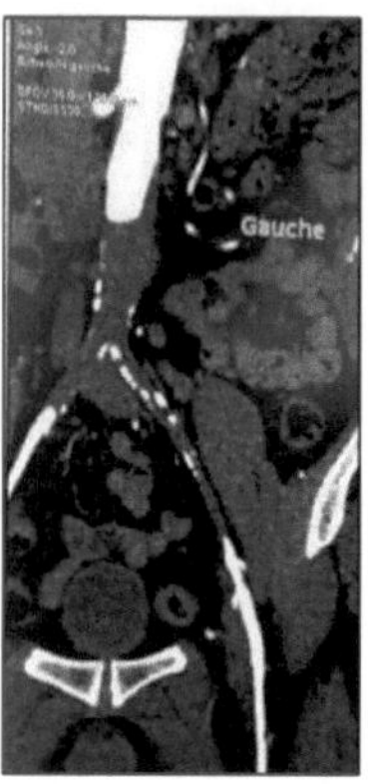

**Figure 1:** Angioscan showing thrombosis of the aortic fork.

## 3- Angio-MRI :

This is a non-invasive technique that does not involve arterial puncture, exposure to X-rays or injection of iodinated contrast.It generally includes one or more morphological sequences and an angiographic sequence. Morphological sequences are acquired using spin echo or fast gradient echo, with T1 or even T2 weighting. The axial plane is useful for analysing the aortic wall and surrounding tissues, while the frontal and sagittal planes can be used to locate pathology in relation to the renal and digestive arteries and the aortic bifurcation.Magnetic resonance imaging has the advantage of spontaneously avoiding the problems associated with radiation and iodinated contrast products. It is reserved for patients allergic to iodine and those with renal insufficiency.

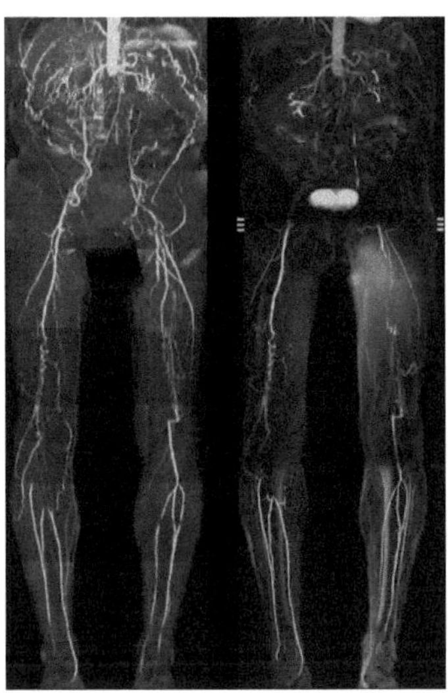

**Figure 2:** Assessment of peripheral arterial disease with magnetic resonance angiography showing bilateral aorto-iliac occlusive disease [29].

## 4- Arteriography :

The artery is approached by percutaneous puncture using the Seldinger technique, then the artery is catheterised using a hydrophilic or teflon-coated guide, allowing a 4 or 5 F valve introducer to be inserted. The probes have an internal lumen for injecting the contrast agent into the catheterised vessel. The material is advanced under fluoroscopic control.An automatic contrast medium injector is needed to allow a flow of extension of the limb homolateral to the arterial puncture for a time proportional to the size of the equipment used. Arteriography provides a map of the arterial tree from the aorta and iliac arteries to the feet. It is used to locate stenoses and occlusions. It shows collaterality, the condition of arteries upstream and downstream of lesions, and the condition of renal and visceral arteries [30].

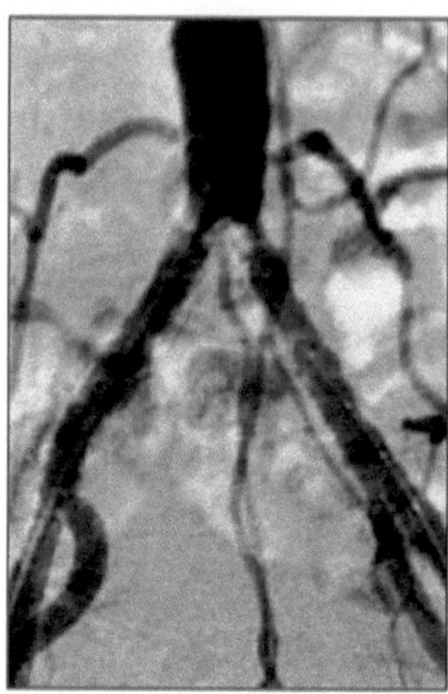

**Figure 3:** Digitised arteriogram showing a bilateral calcified stenotic lesion at the origin of the primitive iliac arteries [31].

However, it is no longer used for diagnostic purposes, but still has a role to play in pre-therapy, particularly in interventional procedures. The limitations of angiography are essentially the lack of direct analysis of the arterial wall and its environment.

# V- TREATMENT

## 1- Medical treatment :

The HAS recommended that all patients with asymptomatic or symptomatic peripheral arterial disease should be treated with a combination of a converting enzyme inhibitor, a statin and an anti-platelet agent [32].

Regular walking training also improves symptoms, with an increase in patients' walking perimeter [33].

Controlling risk factors is also important: stopping smoking and strict control of blood sugar levels according to the guidelines of the American Diabetes Associations are of paramount importance [34].

Hypertension should be controlled according to the recommendations of the Joint National Committee VII, and cholesterol levels according to those of the National Cholesterol Education Program Adult Treatment Panel III [35].

## 2- Surgical treatment :

The two classic methods of surgical treatment of aorto-iliac occlusive lesions are thromboendarterectomy and aorto-bifemoral or aorto-bi-iliac bypass. Extra-anatomical axillofemoral and axillobifemoral bypasses are an alternative surgical technique described in 1966 by Blaisdell and Hall [36].

## 2- 1- Pre-operative assessment :

- **Assessment of cardiac status:** The association of arteriopathy of the lower limbs and atheroma of the coronary arteries is fairly frequent. A coronary assessment is therefore essential before the operation, and should include a clinical examination, questioning and a resting ECG. Thallium myocardial scintigraphy is a good alternative to stress testing. Echocardiography detects abnormalities in myocardial contraction, areas of akinesia indicative of previous infarctions and any associated valvular anomalies. If these tests are positive, coronary angiography is indicated.

- **Assessment of the supra-aortic trunks:** The combination of arteriopathy of the lower limbs and damage to the cerebral vessels is less common than coronary artery disease, but should not be underestimated.

The search for damage to the supra-aortic trunks includes a neurological examination, a search for a transient ischaemic attack, and a systematic ultrasound Doppler of the supra-aortic trunks.

- **Assessment of digestive vessels:** The search for mesenteric involvement is assessed by pre-operative angio-scanner.

- **Assessment of renal function:** Stenosis of the renal artery should be suspected in hypertensive patients or those with renal insufficiency. Questioning and laboratory tests are the basis of this investigation. Renal ultrasound and Doppler ultrasound of the renal arteries should be performed if there is the slightest doubt.

- **Assessment of respiratory function:** A pre-operative assessment of respiratory function is necessary, given the frequency of respiratory complications in smokers and when a trans-peritoneal approach is used.

## 2- 2- Surgical revascularisation techniques :

Conventional open surgery is based on aorto-iliac or aorto-femoral bypass surgery, aorto-iliac endarterectomy and extra-anatomical bypass surgery [37, 38].

- **Endarterectomy:** Endarterectomy is one of the oldest techniques in vascular surgery. It was introduced in 1946 by Dos Santos, who was the first to perform an endarterectomy to treat an occlusive lesion of the superficial femoral artery [39].

In 1951, Wylie was the first to perform an endarterectomy of the aorto-iliac segment [40].Le Veen [40] was the first to describe the technique of semi-closed retroperitoneal endarterectomy in 1965. He described the manual removal of atherosclerotic plaque by means of short arteriotomies of the aorta and iliac arteries and using an arterial unblocking device [40, 41].

 This technique takes into account the three-layer organisation of the artery wall and the possibility of cleaving the lesions using a spatula, generally in the plane of the external elastic boundary located at the level of the outer third of the media.A gently sloping end to the endarterectomy plaque, with no intimal protrusion, is essential to prevent immediate or early thrombo-embolic complications. The absence of residual stenosis after direct closure of the arteriotomy is the most effective way of preventing restenosis in the medium or long term. For this reason, it is preferable to close over a prosthetic or venous widening patch.

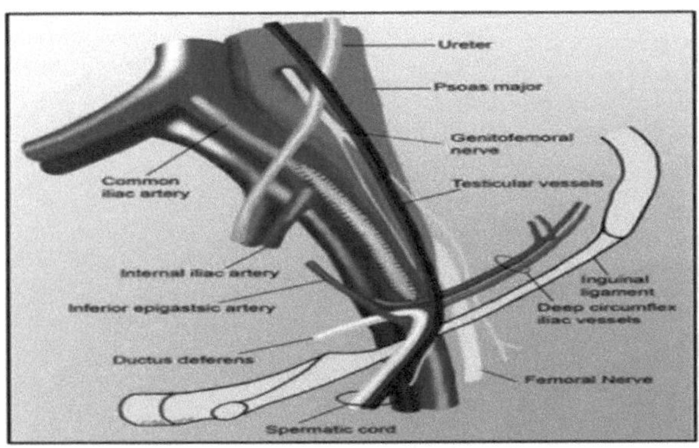


**Figure 4:** Illustration of external iliac artery endarterectomy with patch enlargement [42].

Endarterectomy is most often performed on short lesions that are fully exposed by an arteriotomy centred on the lesion. Endarterectomy may be performed as an adjunct to bypass surgery.

- **Revascularisation by bypass grafts:** The aim of bypass grafts is to create a bypass by directing blood from a healthy area located upstream of the atherosclerotic lesion to another healthy area located downstream in an area affected by ischaemia.

There are two types of bypass: anatomical or extra-anatomical.

The availability of Dacron aorto-femoral and aorto-bifemoral bypasses made it possible to replace endarterectomy techniques in the 1970s [43].

When the operation is limited to an aorto-femoral or aorto-iliac bypass, a trans-peritoneal or retroperitoneal approach is used. The retroperitoneal approach: The incision begins on the midline, two fingerbreadths below the umbilicus and is directed towards the tip of the 11$^{\text{ème}}$ rib, which it extends 3 cm beyond.

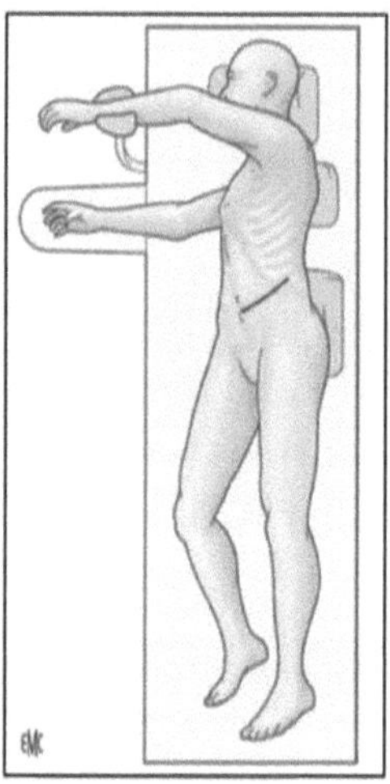

**Figure 5:** Rob's retroperitoneal approach: skin incision from the midline to the tip of the 11$^{\text{ème}}$ rib [44].

Once the muscular layers have been opened, the abdominal aorta and iliac vessels are exposed after the peritoneum has been detached [44].

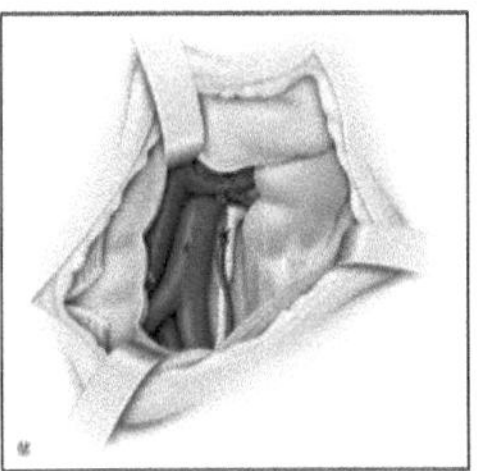

**Figure 6:** Exposure of the aorta and iliac arteries using the retroperitoneal approach [44].

The retroperitoneal approach to the aorta is associated with fewer pulmonary complications and fewer stays in intensive care units than the transperitoneal approach [45]. Transperitoneal approach: The patient lies supine, with a transverse rod under the lumbar region. The surgeon is positioned on the patient's left, with two assistants opposite. This approach can be made either by a median incision from the xiphoid appendix to the sub-subumbilical (xipho-pubic), or by a transverse incision involving only the two rectus muscles.

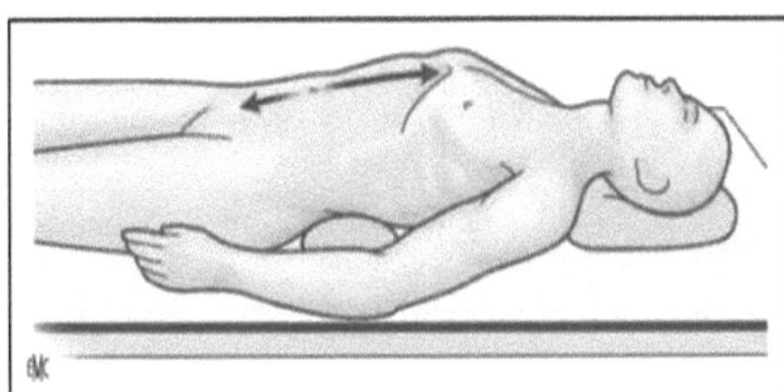

**Figure 7:** Median xiphopubic laparotomy approach [44].

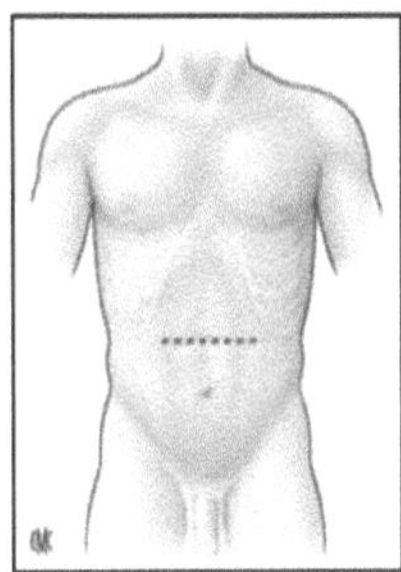

**Figure 8:** Transverse laparotomy respecting the broad abdominal muscles [44].

The transperitoneal route has the advantage of simplicity. It allows complete visceral exploration and an associated visceral procedure, and makes it easier to revascularise the internal iliac artery, inferior mesenteric artery, renal artery and superior mesenteric artery beyond the first six centimetres. However, it is associated with a non-negligible rate of secondary parietal complications such as ventration and respiratory complications.Extension towards the femoral tripods is achieved very simply by means of a separate incision in Scarpa's triangle. The operation begins with a complete visceral exploration, followed by a latero-duodenal incision of the posterior parietal peritoneum.The duodeno-jejunal angle is unhooked. The lower edge of the left renal vein is then marked, which usually forms the upper limit of the dissection. The peritoneal incision is continued downwards as far as the iliac, taking care to avoid the ureteral pedicle. The primitive iliac artery can then be checked separately, respecting the roots of the presacral nerve, and then possibly the branches of this artery: the external iliac artery and the hypogastric artery.Proximal extension to control the inter-renal aorta and renal arteries may require mobilisation or sectioning of the left renal vein.A proximal extension to control the supra-celiac aorta is easily achieved through the same midline incision.Disobstruction of the juxta-renal aorta requires control of the supra-renal aorta. This can be performed either at the level of the supra-celiac aorta, or immediately above the renal arteries. Once the supra-renal clamp has been fitted and the arteriotomy performed, the thrombus and atheromatous debris are precisely removed under visual control. The choice between a proximal anastomosis from the end-to-end or end-to-side sub-renal aorta is controversial. End-to-end anastomosis allows the aorta and prosthesis to meet congruently, so there is no competition with the iliac axes. Peritonisation and isolation of the prosthesis from the duodenal framework is facilitated, thereby reducing the incidence of prosthetic-digestive fistulas. The disadvantages of this method are that it exposes patients to an additional risk of erectile dysfunction, and that it only ensures retrograde revascularisation of the underlying aortic segment and internal iliac arteries. However, termino-terminal anastomosis is technically more difficult in the presence of posterior calcified plaques requiring very high aortic clamping. In contrast, end-to-side anastomosis is technically simpler to perform, and enables direct flow to be maintained in all the arterial branches arising from the sub-renal aorta.

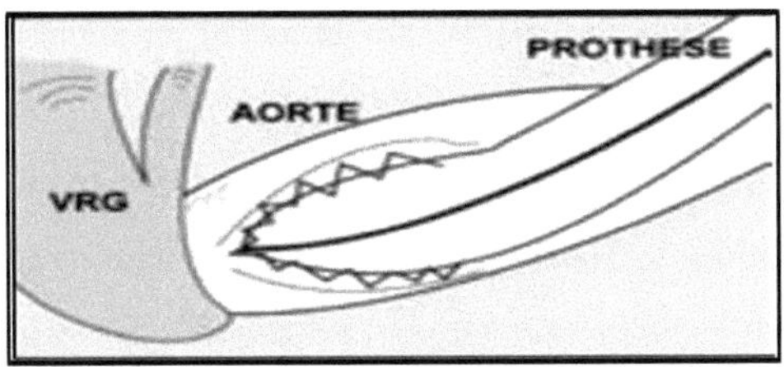


**Figure 9:** Intraoperative view of an endolateral prosthetic aortic anastomosis [46].

Consequently, it reduces the incidence of erectile dysfunction and colonic ischaemia. However, it exposes the patient to turbulence, to plication of the branches at their origin, and to prosthetic-digestive fistulas [47]. Aorto-biliac bypass avoids all the complications associated with a Scarpa's triangle approach: lymphorrhoea, prosthetic infection, and false prosthetic-femoral anastomotic aneurysm. Aorto-bifemoral bypass is necessary in cases of lesions of the external iliac artery. It may be combined with deep plasty in cases of ostial stenosis of the deep femoral artery, or with endarterectomy of the femoral tripod.

**- Associated revascularisation of the renal arteries:** Aorto-iliac atheromatous occlusion is frequently associated with lesions of the renal arteries.

Traditionally, renal artery reconstructions have been performed in patients with symptomatic disease, such as hypertension resistant to medical treatment, or renal failure, associated with haemodynamically significant renal artery stenosis. Renal artery reconstructive surgery for concomitant asymptomatic renal artery stenosis in patients undergoing aortic reconstruction for repair of aneurysm or aorto-iliac occlusive disease is more controversial [48]. The rationale for such an aggressive policy is centred on published data on the natural history of renal artery stenosis. Schreiber et al [49] reported angiographic data of renal arteries showing disease progression in 44% of cases. Thirty-nine percent of stenoses greater than 75% were occluded over time, while only 5% of lesions less than 50% were occluded. Zierler et al [50] documented an annual occlusion rate of 5% for renal artery lesions greater than 60%. Similarly, 4 other retrospective studies that used angiography over a 10-year period demonstrated an overall progression rate of 36% to 53%, often in association with reduced renal function [49, 51]. Studies have shown that surgical procedures for renal preservation and stabilisation have minimised the long-term use of dialysis in these patients [51, 52, 53, 54, 55].

**- Associated revascularisation of the digestive arteries:** It is currently accepted that any stenosis of more than 70% of the superior mesenteric artery represents a high risk of early post-operative digestive ischaemic complications [56]. Aorto-mesenteric bypass combined with aorto-bifemoral bypass or aortic endarterectomy considerably increases the operating time, but may prevent post-operative mesenteric infarction [57].

**- Revascularisation of associated femoropopliteal lesions:** A double-stage revascularisation procedure is indicated when there are associated significant femoropopliteal lesions in critically ischaemic patients.

**- Extra-anatomical bypasses:** Introduced by Freeman and Leeds in 1952, these are defined as bypasses that leave a complete or partial arterial obliteration in place and revascularise the arterial axis downstream of it by a bypass that does not follow the anatomical path of the native arterial axis [58]. These procedures are most often used for lesions of the

aorto-iliac junction and the iliac axes [59]. These bypasses are characterised by their technical simplicity and low surgical aggression. Their use should only be reserved for patients at high surgical risk, or with a hostile abdomen or a history of prosthetic infection preventing direct aorto-iliac surgery. These revascularisations are represented by axillofemoral or axillibifemoral bypasses, and crossed femorofemoral bypasses in the case of unilateral iliac lesions.

- **Laparoscopic minimally invasive surgery:** Laparoscopy is a minimally invasive surgical technique for diagnosis and intervention, which involves accessing the abdominal cavity without opening the abdominal wall. It reduces the surgical aggression caused by abdominal or lumbar incisions. The aim is to treat aorto-iliac lesions with a patency rate of over 90% at 5 years, while benefiting from the advantages of minimally invasive surgery, in particular the reduction in surgical trauma. Dion described the first video-assisted aorto-bifemoral bypass in 1993 [60].

In the past, the Swan Ganz catheter was used to estimate blood volume reliably. This has now been replaced by trans-oesophageal echocardiography, which can be used to detect haemodynamic changes and myocardial perfusion in order to reduce cardiovascular mortality and morbidity [61]. Ultrasound provides a better assessment of left ventricular load by estimating ventricular volumes, and also allows analysis of the segmental kinetics of the left ventricular wall and therefore early and sensitive detection of myocardial ischaemia, which is manifested by more or less extensive dyskinesia or akinesia.

Assessment of myocardial contractility and blood volume by trans-oesophageal echocardiography should therefore be used more widely in patients with a history of heart disease in order to optimise their intra- and post-operative management; alternatively, monitoring via a catheter in the pulmonary artery is indicated for certain patients selected after pre-operative assessment. In 1996, Berens et al [62] published the first series of 4 cases of video-assisted surgery for aorto-iliac occlusive disease. In the same year, Dion et al [63] described the first 2 cases of laparoscopic aorto-bifemoral bypass surgery for aorto-iliac occlusive disease. As with conventional surgery, laparoscopic aorto-iliac surgery can be performed transperitoneally or retroperitoneally [64]. The particularities of laparoscopy compared with open surgery are: the technically demanding procedure, the creation of the pneumoperitoneum, the placement of trocars through 5 to 10 mm incisions, and the use of specific instruments. The patient is positioned in a 45° lateral decubitus position, allowing the digestive tract to move naturally to the right under the effect of gravity, freeing up the area of access to the aorta. A first trocar is introduced into the left flank and a pneumoperitoneum is insufflated, creating a large intra-abdominal working space. A laparoscope fitted with a camera is introduced into the abdomen. Two trocars are inserted close to the midline and the instruments used for dissection are introduced. The aorta is approached in the retroperitoneum. It is checked and clamped.The main difficulty with totally laparoscopic aortic restorations lies in making the arterial anastomosis.

- **Results of laparoscopic surgery:** Laparoscopic surgery offers a number of advantages: less post-operative pain as the abdominal opening is reduced, fewer post-operative cardiac and respiratory complications, shorter hospital stays and a quicker return to normal life. This technique, which has undergone a number of technical improvements, is designed to offer patients revascularisation of the heart and lung. as effective as that carried out by conventional means with minimal invasiveness, has shown promising results in terms of efficacy and safety [65].


## 2-3- Endovascular treatment :

Percutaneous treatment of obstructive lesions of the aorto-iliac junction is currently a safe alternative in terms of morbidity, mortality and patency. It avoids the need for laparotomy and its associated complications. Endovascular techniques now play an important role in the treatment of AOMI [37]. Indeed, trends in the treatment of aorto-iliac occlusive disease have changed. Rates of aorto-femoral bypass surgery have fallen, while the use of angioplasty and stenting of the iliac artery has increased [66]. Recent studies of endovascular treatment of the most severe cases of aorto-iliac occlusive disease have shown results approaching those of open surgery [67]. Several techniques, whose long-term results remain uneven, are currently proposed: - Balloon angioplasty: This consists of restoring a sufficient diameter to the arterial lumen by inflation of a balloon introduced via a guide by remote arterial puncture (usually via the femoral artery) and positioned in contact with the atherosclerotic lesion. Single balloon angioplasty using the kissing balloon technique is used by most authors to treat short (less than 2 cm), concentric, non-calcified stenoses of the aorto-iliac junction [68]. Simultaneous inflation of the angioplasty balloons, placed at the level of the aorto-iliac junction, from each of the primitive iliac arteries, avoids the complications encountered in unilateral angioplasties, such as embolisation or contralateral iliac compression [69].

Angioplasty with stenting: advances in endovascular techniques and instruments have made it possible to extend the range of recanalisation options during treatment of chronic iliac occlusions [70]. The indications for stenting given in the literature are recanalisation of occlusions of the subrenal aorta and the aortic bifurcation, failure and complications of balloon angioplasty, and complex lesions.The technical success rate for this procedure is only around 80% [71]. However, the use of re-entry systems has improved the results of these procedures. Studies have suggested that long-term patency rates approach those of the gold standard of aortofemoral bypass [72]. Jacobs et al [73] reported the largest series with 20 iliac occlusions recanalised using a re-entry device and a 100% success rate. The meta-analysis by Bosch [72] showed that the initial technical success of aorto-iliac stenting was superior to that of simple balloon stenting (96% versus 91%), with identical mortality and morbidity rates, and that stenting reduced the risk of long-term failure by 39% compared with simple balloon stenting. In the series by Kashyap et al [67], 86 patients were randomised to bifemoral bypass surgery and 83 to percutaneous revascularisation. The authors concluded that percutaneous revascularisation is a suitable and less invasive alternative to anatomical surgical revascularisation for the treatment of severe aortoiliac lesions.

## 3- Indications:

The therapeutic strategy must be adapted to the patient's general condition, and to the morphology and extent of the lesions and the downstream bed, as well as to the personal experience of the practitioners caring for these patients.

### - ACC (American College of Cardiology) and AHA (American Heart Association) recommendations:

There has been a change in indications over the last 25 years, with the treatment of aorto-iliac occlusive disease moving from open surgery by aorto-biliac or aorto-bi-femoral bypass to endovascular treatments for diffuse diseases (TASC D). This preference for less invasive techniques is based on evidence and driven by a shorter length of stay (or entirely outpatient treatment) and a reduction in peri-operative morbidity and mortality, while achieving comparable patency (primary patency rates at 4 to 5 years are 60% to 86%, and secondary patency rates are 80% to 98%) [74].

**- ESC recommendations [75]:** The recommendations issued by the ESC (European Society of Cardiology) are based solely on lesion criteria. These recommendations are :

- When revascularisation is indicated, initial endovascular treatment is recommended for TASC A, B and C aortoiliac lesions.

- A primary endovascular approach may be considered for TASC D aortoiliac lesions in patients with severe co-morbidities, in experienced teams.

- Primary stenting is preferable to selective stenting in the case of an aorto-iliac lesion.

**Recommendations for revascularization in patients with aortoiliac lesions**

| Recommendations | Class[a] | Level[b] |
| --- | --- | --- |
| When revascularization is indicated, an endovascular-first strategy is recommended in all aortoiliac TASC A–C lesions. | I | C |
| A primary endovascular approach may be considered in aortoiliac TASC D lesions in patients with severe comorbidities, if done by an experienced team. | IIb | C |
| Primary stent implantation rather than provisional stenting may be considered for aortoiliac lesions. | IIb | C |

[a]Class of recommendation.
[b]Level of evidence.
TASC = TransAtlantic Inter-Society Consensus.

**Figure 10:** Recommendations for revascularisation of aorto-iliac lesions [75].

Despite the relative absence of data evaluating its long-term results, these recommendations give endovascular treatment of arteriopathy a large place. In 2011, the European Society of Cardiology (ESC) [76] and the ACC guidelines / AHA PAD [77] have recommended a primary endovascular approach for aortoiliac lesions. Borderline lesions should be assessed with haemodynamic gradients and treated with primary stenting [78].

The Bravissimo study [79], which evaluated the results of vascular stents in the treatment of iliac lesions in 325 patients with TASC A, B, C and D lesions, showed 100% technical success with a primary patency rate at 24 months of 87.9%.

**- TASC II recommendations for aorto-iliac lesions [80]:** According to the TASCII classification of aorto-iliac occlusive disease, lesions can be classified as type A, B, C or D, with type A representing short segmental stenosis of the common or external iliac artery. Lesions increase in complexity with type B, then type C, and finally with type D representing long-segment occlusions of the common and external iliac arteries.

According to TASC II recommendations, endovascular therapy is the preferred treatment method for type A lesions. Surgery is preferred for type D lesions. Some patients with type B and C lesions may be managed with surgery or endovascular therapy, depending on the informed patient's choice, medical co-morbidities and the surgeon's experience [80].

In the case of associated lesions of the femoropopliteal axis, some studies have shown that simultaneous femoropopliteal bypass surgery is indicated regardless of the clinical stage, since it increases the long-term patency of an aortic prosthesis [81].

# VI- RESULTS OF SURGICAL TREATMENT

Surgery improves patients' functional quality of life by saving limbs.

## 1- Extra-anatomical bypasses :

The results for extra-anatomical bypasses (axillofemoral or femorofemoral) are not as good as those for aortofemoral or aortoiliac bypasses.Operative mortality is between 0 and 4% for femoral-femoral bypass, and between 2 and 11% for axillary-bifemoral bypass [29]. The study by Liedenbaum MH et al [82] found a 30-day mortality rate of 17%. This rate is much higher than the rate found in a similar study by Martin and Katz, which was 4.9% [83]. Schneider et al [84] described a 30-day mortality rate of 18% in their axillofemoral bypass group.These high mortality rates may be explained by the fact that the patients in the axillofemoral bypass group were older and had more major risk factors than the patients who underwent aorto-bifemoral bypass. The 5-year primary patency rate for extra-anatomical bypass surgery for aorto-iliac occlusive disease is 19-50% for axillobifemoral bypass and 44-85% for femorofemoral bypass [29]. The study by Liedenbaum MH and Verdam FJ found a primary patency rate of 49% at 3 years [82]. The patency rate at 3 years was 72% in the study by Martin and Katz, and 63% in the study by Schneider et al [83, 84]. Olson et al [85] examined the results of axillofemoral bypass surgery performed as a treatment for failure of the initial anatomical revascularisation. At 18 months, the patency rate of these extra-anatomical bypasses was 54%.

## 2- Anatomical bypasses :

The aortic bypass procedure is associated with a significant post-operative risk due to the complexity of surgical and medical complications. Mortality is due not only to peripheral damage, but also to other sites of atheromatous disease, particularly coronary and cerebral. This explains the operative mortality rate in recent series of around 2.7% for aorto-femoral bypass surgery [86]. Anidjar et al [87] reported a mortality rate of less than 3% after 385 anatomical aortic restorations performed for occlusive lesions.Based on data from more than 3,500 bifurcated aortic bypass procedures, this study showed that during the first 30 days, 3.6% of patients died and approximately one fifth experienced a major complication [88].Bifurcated aortic bypass surgery should therefore be considered a high-risk procedure and requires meticulous pre-operative assessment whenever an endovascular option is ruled out.Most studies have shown that cardiac causes are at the top of the list for mortality in patients with arterial disease, accounting for more than 50% of deaths in the immediate post-operative period. Renal failure is also a major cause of peri-operative mortality. Indeed, renal artery damage has been observed in up to 29% of patients with chronic aorto-iliac occlusive disease. Because of this association with disease, early studies suggested that simultaneous repair should be performed if the patient presented an appropriate surgical risk. This approach would simplify patient management and avoid secondary surgery and the need for multiple administration of anaesthesia. However, these combined procedures have historically carried higher rates of morbidity and mortality.

The 1975 Renovascular Hypertension Cooperative Study found a mortality rate of 25% in patients undergoing combined procedures. Additional recent reports have demonstrated peri-operative mortality rates of 2% to 6% [89, 90, 53].

In the series by R. Clement Darling [49], if patients undergoing emergent aortic repair are separated from those undergoing elective aortic repair with concomitant renal artery reconstruction, the operative mortality rate is not statistically different from that of patients undergoing aortic repair alone. Anatomical revascularisation surgery from the abdominal aorta exposes patients to specific complications, such as myocardial and mesenteric ischaemia, and renal failure. Other complications arise from laparotomy, such as respiratory complications.

Cardiac complications, whether acute coronary insufficiency, heart failure or rhythm disorders, are a major cause of mortality after abdominal aortic surgery [62].

The rate of post-operative infarction is currently less than 3%. Diagnostic methods for post-operative ischaemic cardiac complications are based on the clinic, analysis of the electrocardiogram, trans-thoracic echocardiography and measurement of plasma troponin levels.The study by Bredahl and Jensen [88] found a cardiac complication rate of 6%, and 30% of patients with a cardiac complication died within the first 30 days following anatomical aorto-iliac revascularisation.Respiratory complications may include infectious pneumonitis, atelectasis with bronchial congestion, or acute respiratory failure. Rigorous physiotherapy combined with effective analgesia could improve respiratory status.According to the study by Bredahl and Jensen [88], pulmonary complications were the most frequent medical complications. Nearly 10% of their patients suffered from pneumonia or respiratory distress syndrome or required prolonged mechanical ventilation. However, this rate is lower than the 13% to 16% rate of major pulmonary complications reported in other studies [91].Neurological complications are dominated by stroke. In exceptional cases, spinal cord ischaemia may occur. The risk of stroke after revascularisation surgery using the abdominal aorta is estimated at 1%. This is usually a complication related to undiagnosed preoperative tight stenosis of the internal carotid artery.In a report of 1390 patients undergoing non-carotid vascular operations, including aortic reconstruction and limb bypass surgery The overall incidence of stroke or transient ischaemic attack was 0.9% [92].

Spinal cord ischaemia is an exceptional complication of aortic surgery performed under sub-renal clamping [93]. In the few cases reported in the literature, it seems to be the consequence of a distal embolism, either of an interruption in the vascularisation of the lumbosacral branches of the internal iliac arteries, or of an abnormal birth of Adamkiewicz's artery. The risk factors are supra-renal clamping, prolonged aortic clamping, intra-operative arterial hypotension, absence of systemic heparinisation prior to clamping, and above all end-to-end aortic anastomosis.Digestive complications are the most frequent complications arising after abdominal aortic surgery. Mesenteric ischaemia is one of the most serious complications following abdominal aortic surgery. In the initial phase, the clinical examination is often poor, with no indication of any specific clinical signs. The abdominal syndrome consists mainly of mild signs of obstruction, sometimes with an early resumption of transit through fetid or bloody diarrhoea.Post-operative colonoscopy is used to determine the extent and intensity of the lesions. Intensive resuscitation must be associated with the surgical procedure, which has two components:

- A vascular flap, either by bypass surgery or, in the event of an embolism, by deobstruction.

- An intestinal component consisting of resection of the necrotic intestinal loops and restoration of digestive continuity.

If the ischaemia is not too severe and is reversible, only revascularisation is necessary.

In Kim Bredahl's study, which included all patients who had undergone biiliac or aorto-bifemoral bypass surgery in Denmark from 1993 to 2012, the incidence of mesenteric ischaemia was 1.6% [88].

Post-operative ileus is common after abdominal aortic surgery. Transit is usually resumed by $2^{\text{ème}}$ or $3^{\text{ème}}$ days post-operatively in the case of a retroperitoneal approach, and between $3^{\text{ème}}$ and $5^{\text{ème}}$ days in the case of a transperitoneal approach.Published data from randomised studies have suggested that the incidence of paralytic ileus varies from 7% to 10% after trans-peritoneal operations [94, 95]. The incidence of ileus is lower after retroperitoneal operations.Early bypass thrombosis is a serious complication which may occur immediately on awakening from surgery or in the hours or days following the operation. The rate of this complication varies from one series to another, ranging from 1.4% to 8.3% [96, 97].The incidence of early occlusion of bifurcated aortic bypass was 1.9% in the series by Kim Bredhal [88].

Clinically, thrombosis often manifests itself as acute ischaemia, ranging from coldness to cyanosis and sensory-motor disorders of the limb(s) in question. Sometimes thrombosis is asymptomatic, in which case the diagnosis is confirmed by pulse examination and post-operative Doppler.Once the diagnosis has been made, the patient must undergo a procedure to remove the blockage, sometimes involving repair of the anastomoses. Early postoperative haemorrhage is a common complication of aorto-iliac surgery. It occurs in 2-6% of cases [88, 98].The main causes of post-operative bleeding are :

- Haemostasis disorders secondary to heparin overdose or drug-induced coagulopathy. Treatment consists of correcting the biological factors. Re-operation is necessary in the event of a large haematoma leading to consumption of coagulation factors.

- Surgical bleeding from a vascular wound or anastomotic dehiscence.

To prevent post-operative bleeding, a pre-operative haemostasis check-up is necessary, and caution during the operation is recommended, with checks to ensure that the anastomoses are watertight and that the operation is performed with care to avoid injury to the iliac veins.

In the absence of pre-operative renal damage, the occurrence of acute renal failure in the post-operative period remains a rare event.

However, it can occur as a result of aggravation of pre-existing renal insufficiency.

The main cause of post-operative renal failure is renal hypoperfusion secondary to cardiac failure or hypovolaemia during surgery, especially aortic decompression.It may also be secondary to truncal obliteration of one or both renal arteries by embolism of atheromatous material. Supra-renal aortic clamping is also a factor in post-operative acute renal failure [99].

The mortality rate caused by post-operative acute renal failure is around 1% [88].

The best way to preserve renal function is to maintain a stable haemodynamic state during and after the operation, and to restore blood loss immediately using a transfusion protocol based on haemoglobin level monitoring. Ureteral lesions may be an unrecognised peroperative ureteral wound or localised ureteral necrosis associated with extensive devascularisation.These two complications are rare. They lead to a ureteral fistula, which manifests itself as a post-operative discharge of urine through the suction drains.Diagnosis of this fistula is based on intravenous urography, which shows the leakage of opaque product. Treatment of the ureteral lesion is based on retrograde ureteral catheterisation or percutaneous nephrostomy [100].

Complete knowledge of the anatomical relationship of the ureter to the iliac bifurcation is therefore essential. Direct injury to the ureter is best avoided by keeping the dissection close to the arterial wall and dissecting the ureter from the iliac arteries during retroperitoneal tunnelling. Sexual dysfunction after aorto-iliac surgery is associated with a combination of haemodynamic changes in pelvic circulation due to reduced hypogastric flow and interruption of the pre-aortic plexus [101].

The overall incidence of early postoperative prosthetic infections is estimated at 1 to 2%. It is clearly decreasing compared to previous decades due to the generalisation of antibiotic prophylaxis [87].

Early prosthetic infections are most often caused by Staphylococcus aureus and are accompanied by obvious general and local signs. Despite the encouraging long-term results of anatomical revascularisation of aorto-iliac occlusive disease, late complications continue to occur throughout follow-up. The results of the various series have shown that only in exceptional cases do patients die from aorto-iliac atherosclerosis, but more often from another location of atheromatous disease or another pathology, particularly neoplasia. The patency rate of aorto-bifemoral bypasses is 85% at 5 years, between 80 and 90% at 10 years, and 70% at 15 years [102, 103]. Late thrombosis of prostheses is the most frequent late complication. However, the average annual rate of thrombosis is between 2% and 4%, and is currently tending to decrease thanks to improvements in materials and surgical techniques. Thrombosis generally occurs in one of the two dividing branches of an aorto-biliac or aorto-bifemoral bypass. Late thrombosis may be related to the progressive deterioration of the downstream bed as atheromatous disease progresses, especially in patients with uncontrolled atherosclerotic risk factors [104].Treatment of late prosthetic occlusion may involve surgical thrombectomy, revascularisation by extra-anatomical bypass or complete prosthetic replacement:

- Thrombectomy of the prosthesis is the treatment most frequently used by most teams. It is a simple procedure performed under local or local-regional anaesthetic with an approach to the Scarpa.

However, this procedure may lead to contralateral embolisation or weakening of the proximal anastomosis.

- Complete prosthetic replacement, which gives a better long-term result but involves a significant morbidity and mortality rate.

- Extra-anatomical revascularisation: this is a method of treating late obliteration of prosthetic branches when the contralateral branch remains patent.

Cross-femoral bypass may be used as an alternative surgical option if the contralateral iliofemoral arterial axis is free of significant stenosis, and especially if thrombectomy fails or thrombosis is diagnosed late [105, 106]. The thoracic aorta can also be used as a site for proximal anastomosis in repeat surgery [107].

Refraining from treatment is indicated when functional discomfort is minimal and the vitality of the limb is not at risk. False anastomotic aneurysms result from dehiscence of the anastomosis, caused by the difference in compliance between the prosthesis and the native artery over time [108]. They are a serious complication with sometimes fatal consequences.The time to onset varies widely, from a few months to several years. The incidence of this complication is very difficult to assess because they remain asymptomatic for a long time Femoral location is the most frequent, with an incidence of 3 to 6% at this site [108], due to the greater frequency of scarring problems and the mechanical stresses to which the anastomosis is subjected at this level, favoured by flexion-extension movements of the thigh. Akker [109] estimated the risk of false aneurysm at 15 years to be 10% at the aortic anastomosis and 15% at the femoral anastomosis.

The factors contributing to the development of this complication are :

- Excessive tension on the anastomosis due to inadequate length of the prosthesis.

- Poor suture at the anastomotic site.

- The thinness of the arterial wall during endarterectomy.

- Rupture of the suture material due to infection.

Diagnosis of a false femoral aneurysm is usually straightforward because it is often a pulsatile mass of the scarpa. Aortic and iliac aneurysms are often asymptomatic. They progress towards expansion, producing occlusion of the prosthesis or emboli responsible for progressive degradation of the downstream bed; or compression of a nearby intra-abdominal organ (duodenum, ureter, inferior vena cava); or rupture, producing pain and haemorrhage of varying severity. False anastomotic aneurysms must be treated even if they are asymptomatic, because of the risk of rupture and distal embolisation. Surgical repair involves resection of the aneurysm followed by restoration of arterial continuity. Bacteriological samples should always be taken to check for infection.Treatment of these lesions by stent grafting has been proposed by a number of authors. The results of repairing false aneurysms are good, particularly if the repair is carried out on a programmed basis. Late prosthetic infection is a serious complication that can threaten the patient's vital and functional prognosis, and its incidence varies from 1 to 2%. They often occur several years after the initial procedure. Staphylococcus aureus is the germ most frequently implicated. Aguiar et al [108] noted an incidence of prosthesis infection of 2.4% after 10 years of monitoring. These late infections may be responsible for long-term inflammatory reactions, or prosthetic complications such as thrombosis or false anastomotic aneurysms.

Imaging can be used to find arguments in favour of :

- A large collection at a distance from the operation, with a thickened, irregular wall enhanced by injection of contrast medium, or a pre-suppurative state with infiltration of the retroperitoneal fat.

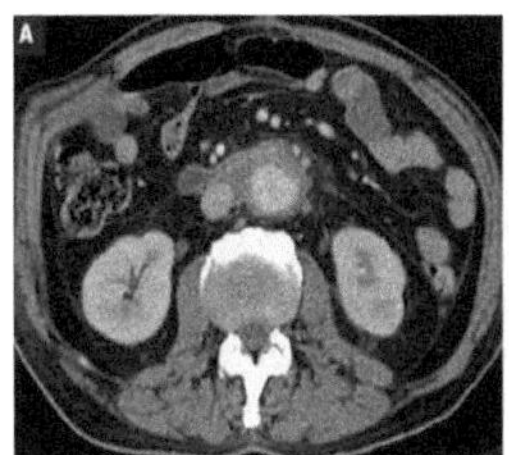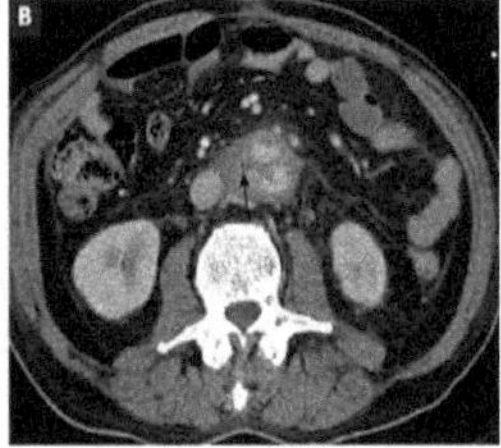

**Figure 11:** Angioscan showing an aortic prosthesis infection: a periprosthetic collection with infiltration of periaortic fat [110].

- Signs that may indicate a fissured state: irregularity of the contour of an anastomosis or an image of addition after opacification.

-An adjacent infectious site within a digestive structure (aorto-enteric fistula, sigmoiditis).

Treatment of these infections involves extensive antibiotic therapy, with explantation of the prosthesis, and restoration of arterial continuity, which can be ensured by :

- Aortic ligation combined with axillofemoral revascularisation is associated with a high rate of reinfection and prosthetic thrombosis [111].

- In situ revascularisation using biological material (arterial allograft) or prosthetic material (prosthesis impregnated with a rifampicin-based antibiotic solution).

Cryopreserved arterial allografts, which have shown satisfactory long-term results, are the material of choice for in situ restorations in cases of prosthetic infection [112].

In cases where the infection is localised, local measures such as local irrigation with antibiotic therapy, drainage and debridement may be sufficient. Prosthetic-digestive fistulas account for 1% of complications of abdominal aortic prostheses, and occur with an average delay of several years. They are the most serious complications of prosthetic infections. The death rate is as high as 70% [113].Their pathogenesis involves mechanical factors of erosion and infectious factors. The intestinal segment most often involved is the distal part of the duodenum (0.5 to 2.4% of cases), but it may also involve an ileal or jejunal loop, the right colon, the left colon, or even the appendix [114].

The diagnosis of a prosthetic-digestive fistula is based on a number of factors:

- Digestive haemorrhage is the main symptom.

- Fever is also a frequent symptom. The presence of a severe late-onset septic syndrome is highly suggestive of a prosthetic-digestive fistula rather than prosthetic sepsis without a fistula.

- Epigastric pain.

Diagnosis is based on digestive endoscopy, which looks for a parietal ulcer of the duodenum, and abdominal helical CT scanning. The CT scan must include a study without injection or ingestion of contrast agent, then a series after vascular opacification in order to search for passage of contrast agent from the aortic lumen to the digestive lumen, and a series after ingestion of contrast agent in order to search for extravasation of contrast agent from the digestive lumen to the periaortic space [115].Treatment involves three stages: control of haemorrhage and resection of the infected prosthesis, repair of the intestinal lesion, and arterial revascularisation. Digestive repair should be carried out prior to revascularisation whenever possible in order to eliminate contamination of the replacement material. Arterial continuity is re-established either by arterial allograft or by an extra-anatomical axillofemoral or axillobifemoral bypass graft to avoid infectious complications associated with the prosthesis in place [116].Regardless of the revascularisation technique chosen, the results are poorer than for sepsis without a digestive fistula. The possible causes of death are rupture of the aortic stump in the case of extra-anatomical revascularisation, and recurrence of the fistula in the case of in situ revascularisation. Late urological complications are dominated by pyelo-caliceal dilatations, which are fairly frequent in the immediate aftermath of aortic surgery. If they persist, the obstruction must be removed. Obstruction may be due to reactive scar fibrosis where the ureter crosses the prosthesis, or to tunnelling of the prosthesis in front of the ureter, which is compressed between the prosthesis and the native arterial axis. Sexual problems may manifest themselves as erectile dysfunction or ejaculation problems secondary to a section of the presacral nerves.

# VII- CONCLUSION

The treatment of aorto-iliac occlusive lesions is evolving rapidly. Multiple approaches need to be considered, ranging from medical management to surgical and endovascular procedures.The development of endovascular techniques, resulting in increased procedural success, reduced complications and increased long-term patency, continues to reduce the role of surgery, particularly for short aorto-iliac lesions.Trends in the treatment of aorto-iliac occlusive disease have therefore changed. Rates of bypass surgery from the aorta are falling, while the use of angioplasty and stenting is increasing.However, anatomical restorative surgery from the sub-renal abdominal aorta is a proven treatment for the management of aorto-iliac occlusive disease.Patients who are candidates for this type of surgery pose a number of different problems. In the pre-operative period, the main concern is to assess the operative risk. Intra-operatively, the choice of anaesthetic technique is essential, as is rigorous haemodynamic monitoring. Finally, the post-operative period is marked by a risk of cardiac and respiratory complications, as well as specific complications that need to be diagnosed early.The clinical symptoms of aorto-iliac atherosclerosis are dominated by intermittent claudication. However, atherosclerosis may be discovered in the presence of trophic disorders, decubitus pain or signs of acute arterial occlusion.The morphological and topographical study of these lesions is now well established thanks to ultrasound and CT scanning of the arterial axes.Pre-operative assessment is an important part of the therapeutic strategy. Its aim is to reduce peri-operative morbidity and mortality, thereby improving long-term survival. Given the frequent association between atheromatous coronary and carotid lesions and arteriopathy of the lower limbs, and the significant postoperative morbidity and mortality, a coronary and carotid work-up is essential in all patients proposed for anatomical revascularisation using the abdominal aorta. The development of endovascular treatment techniques has simplified the treatment of arterial occlusive lesions. However, anatomical revascularisation from the sub-renal abdominal aorta remains the reference treatment for lesions classified as TASC C and D. Surgery at the aorto-iliac level has a relatively high mortality rate of around 2.7%, due to the frequency of associated coronary and carotid disease [86].

Early morbidity is essentially represented by cardiac complications such as acute coronary insufficiency, heart failure or cardiac rhythm disorders; digestive and cerebral ischaemic complications; and bypass thrombosis. Early bypass thrombosis is an uncommon complication, affecting between 1.4% and 8.4% of patients [96, 97]. The main causes are technical faults and insufficient downstream bed.Late mortality is mainly linked to other sites of atheromatous disease, particularly cardiac, and to neoplastic causes. Patients with aorto-iliac occlusive disease undergoing aorto-bifemoral bypass surgery should be monitored regularly for life after surgery to reduce the risk of prosthetic failure due to aorto-femoral occlusion.progression of atherosclerotic disease or the development of a late anastomotic aneurysm. These patients also have a high rate of distal anastomotic stenosis, most often due to myointimal hyperplasia. Late complications are mainly prosthesis infections and false anastomotic aneurysms. Aorto-bi-iliac or bi-femoral restorations have an excellent long-term patency rate, but occlusive complications can occur. False anastomotic aneurysm is a serious complication with sometimes fatal consequences. Late infection of the prosthetic material is also a major complication that can jeopardise the patient's vital and functional prognosis. Its incidence varies from 1 to 2%. Anatomical surgical revascularisation of aorto-iliac atherosclerotic lesions therefore has its own specific indications. The success of this invasive procedure depends above all on conditioning the patient with a complete pre-operative assessment of atherosclerotic disease and rigorous peri-operative monitoring. This makes it possible to detect and save the patient from complications that could jeopardise his or her vital prognosis.

# BIBLIOGRAPHY

[1] Brewster DC. Direct reconstruction for aorto-iliac occlusive disease. In: Rutherford RB ed. Vascular Surgery. Philadelphia: Saunders, 1995. pp 766-794.

[2] Bacourt F, Foster D, Mignon E. Atherosclerosis obliterans of the lower limbs. Encycl Méd Chir, Angéologie 2002; p 19-1510.

[3] Diehm C, Schuster A, Allenberg JR, Darius H, Haberl R, Lange S, et al. High prevalence of peripheral arterial disease and co-morbidity in 6880 primary care patients: cross-sectional study. Atherosclerosis 2004; 172(1):95-105.

[4] Mbanya JC, Motala AN, Sobngwi E et al. Diabetes in Sub-Saharan Africa. Lancet 2010; 375 (9733): 2254-66.

[5] Criqui MH, Fronek A, Barrett-Connor E, Klauber MR, Gabriel S, Goodman D. The prevalence of peripheral arterial disease in a defined population. Circulation 2000; 71: 510-5.

[6] Boccalon H, Lehert P, Mosnier M. Assessment of the prevalence of arteriopathy of the lower limbs in France using the systolic index in a population at vascular risk. J Mal Vasc 2000; 25: 38-46.

[7] Urnal J, Vascu O, Su L. Epidemiology, natural history, risk factors. Journal of Vascular Surgery 2000; 31(1): 5-34.

[8] Reena L, Todd S, Joshua A et al. Secondary prevention and mortality in peripheral artery disease. National Health and Nutrition Examination Study, 1999 to 2004. Circulation 2011.

[9] Cardiovascular risk factors and prevention. Université Médicale Virtuelle Francophone 2009.

[10] Koskas F, Kieffer E. Chronic atheromatous occlusive lesions of the aorta

and lower limbs. Encycl Méd Chir, AKOS Encycl Prat de Méd, 2-0450, Cardiologie Angéologie 1999; 615(11):10.

[11] Price JF, Mowbray PI, Lee AJ, Rumley A, Lowe GD, Fowkes FG. Relationship between smoking and cardiovascular risk factors in the development of peripheral arterial disease and coronary artery disease: Edinburgh Artery Study. Eur Heart J 2001; 20:344-53.

[12] Kannel WB, Mc Gee DL. Update on some epidemiologic features of intermittent claudication: the Framingham Study. J Am Geriatr Soc 2002; 33:13-8.

[13] International Diabetes Federation. Diabetes Atlas 4th edition. Montreal 2009: 22-36.

[14] Hiatt WR, Marshall JA, Baxter J, Hildebrandt W, Kahn LR, Hamman RF et al. Diagnostic methods for peripheral arterial disease in the San Luis Valley Diabetes Study. J Clin Epidemiol 2003; 43:597-606.

[15] Khan N, ChockalinGam R, Campbell N. Lack of control of high blood pressure and treatment recommendations in Canada. Am J Cardiol 2002; 18 (6): 657-61.

[16] Murabito JM, Evans JC, Nieto K, Larson MG, Levy D, Wilson PWF. Prevalence and clinical correlates of peripheral arterial disease in the Framingham Offspring Study. Am Heart J 2002; 143:961-5.

[17] Dawber, Royle T. The Framingham Study: The epidemiology of atherosclerotic disease. Cambridge Mass, Havard University press 1980.

[18] Sabouret P, Cacoub P, Dallongeville J et al. REACH: International prospective observational registry in patients at risk of atherothrombotic events. Results for the French arm at baseline and one year.Arch cardiovasc Dis 2008; 101 (2): 77-8.

[19] Iglesias JI, Hamburger RJ, Feldman L, et al. The natural history of incidental renal artery stenosis in patients with aorto-iliac vascular disease. Am J Med 2000; 109: 642-7.

[20] John E Connolly, M.D, Jack H M Kwaan. Prophylactic Revascularization of the Gut. From the Department of Surgery, University of California at Irvine and the Long Beach Veterans Administration Medical Center, Long Beach, California.

[21] Leschi JP. Abdominal aorta and carotid arteries. In: Kieffer E, Coriat P, Thomas D, Eds. Le Polyvasculaire Athéromateux. Paris: Editions AERCV, 2000; 61-83.

[22] Chiche L. Abdominal aorta and coronary arteries. In: Kieffer E, Coriat P, Thomas D, Eds. Le Polyvasculaire Athéromateux. Paris: Editions AERCV, 2000; 27-59.

[23] Rose GA. The diagnosis of ischaemic heart pain and intermittent claudication in field surveys. Bull World Health Organ 2000; 27:645-58.

[24] TASC II.Inter-society consensus for the management of peripheral arterial disease. Eur J Vasc Endovasc surg 2007; 33.

[25] Carter SA. Indirect sytolic pressures and pulse waves in arterial occlusive diseases of the lower extremities. Circulation 1968; 37: 624-37.

[26] Hirsch AT, Haskal ZJ, Hertzel NR et al. ACC/AHA 2005 practice guidelines for the management of patients with peripheral arterial disease. Circulation 2006; 113 (11): 1474-547.

[27] Schoul JM, Aranand B, Doumercre P et al. Comparison of risk factors in vascopatic angina without significant fixed coronary narrowing and no vascopatic angina. Am J Cardiol, 1986; 37: 199-202.

[28] Quanadli SD, Lacombe P. Cardiovascular imaging (CT, MRI, angiography).

Chapter IX/C pages 1-5.

[29] Khanjan H Nagarsheth, Vincent Lopez Rowe. Aorto-iliac Occlusive Disease. Updated: Aug 21, 2017.Vascular Surgery.

[30] Elias A, Lefebvre D. Imagerie vasculaire : artériopathie des membres. Chapter 8 pp 99111. Edition Masson 1994.

[31] Picquet J, BlinV, Bouyé P, Perdreau G, Thouveny F, Enon B, L'hoste P. Endovascular treatment by "kissing stent" of obliterating lesions of the aorto-iliac carrefour. J Mal Vasc 2005; 30: 163-170.

[32] Management of chronic obliterative atherosclerotic arterial disease of the lower limbs (indications for medication, revascularisation and rehabilitation). Recommendations for clinical practice. Haute Autorité de Santé, April 2006.

[33] Regensteiner JG, Steiner JF, Hiatt WR. Exercise training improve functional status in patients with peripheral arterial disease. J VascSurg 1996; 23: 104-15.

[34] Executive summary. standards of medical care in diabetes. Diabetes Care 2009; 32(Suppl. 1):S6-S12.

[35] Ong HT. The JNC 7 hypertension guidelines. JAMA 2003; 289:2560-2572.
[36] Blaisdell FW, Hall AD. Axillary femoral bypass for lower extremity ischemia. Surgery 1963;54:563.

[37] Schneider PA. Endovascular or open surgery for aorto-iliac occlusive disease? Cardiovasc. Surg 2002; 10: 378-382.
[38] Nogren L, Hiatt WR, Dormandy JA, et al. Inter-society consensus for the management of peripheral arterial disease. IntAngiol 2007; 26: 81-157.

[39] Dos Santos JC. Sur la désobstruction des thromboses arérielles anciennes. Mem Acad Chir (Paris) 1947; 73: 409-411.

[40] Wylie EJ, Kerr E, Davies O. Experimental and clinical experiences with

the use of fascia lata applied as a graft about major arteries after thrombo-endarterectomy and aneurysmorraphy. Surg Gynecol Obstet1951; 93: 257-272.

[41] Le Veen HH, Diaz C, Christoudias G. The post-endarterectomy intimal flap. Arch Surg 1973; 107: 664-668.

[42] Ebaugh JL, Gupta N, Raffetto JD, Roxbury W, Massachusetts B. External iliac artery endarterectomy with single incision patch angioplasty. Ann Vasc Surg 2011; 25: 1165-1169.

[43] Van Vugt R, Kruse R, Sterkenburg S M, Fritschy W M, Moll Frans L. Semi-closed endarterectomy for aorto-iliac occlusive disease. Ann Vasc Surg 2010; 24: 1082-1088.

[44] Ricco J.B, Sessa C. Abdominal aorta and iliac artery approaches. EMC (Elsevier Masson SAS, Paris), Techniques chirurgicales - Chirurgie vasculaire, 43-034-A, 2010.

[45] Ballord JL, Yonemonto H, Killeen JD, Linda L. An interesting approach to the aorta: the retroperitoneal approach. Ann Chir Vasc 2000; 14: 1-5.

[46] Sumio Fukui, Surgical treatment of obliterative arterial disease of the lower limbs today. Presse Med 2004; 33: 1096-8.

[47] Price GE, Turrentine M, Stringfields. Evaluation of end-to-side vs end-to-end proximal anastomosis in aorto-bifemoral bypass. Arch Surg 1982; 117: 1580.

[48] R. Clement Darling, III, Paul B. Kreienberg, Benjamin B. Chang, Philip S. K. Paty, William E. Lloyd, Robert P. Leather, and Dhiraj M. Shah. Outcome of Renal Artery Reconstruction (Analysis of 687 Procedures) Ann Surg. 1999 Oct; 230(4): 524.

[49] Schreiber MJ, Pohl MA, Novick AC. Thenatural history of atherosclerotic and fibrous renal artery disease. Urol Clin North Am 1984; 11: 383-392.

[50] Zierler RE, Bergelin RO, Isaacson JA, et al. Natural history of atherosclerotic renal artery stenosis: a prospective study with duplex ultrasonography. J Vasc Surg 1994; 19: 250- 258.

[51] Hallett JW, Fowl R, O'Brien PC, et al. Renovascular operations in patients with chronic renal insufficiency: do the benefits justify the risks? J Vasc Surg 1987; 5: 622-627.

[52] Reilly JM, Rubin BG, Thompson RW, et al. Revascularization of the solitary kidney: a challenging problem in a high-risk population. Surgery 1996; 120: 732- 737.

[53] Franklin SS, Young JD, Maxwell MH. Operative morbidity and mortality in renovascular disease. JAMA 1975; 231: 1148-1153.

[54] Elmore JR, Ray FS, Dillihunt RC, Herbert WE. Renal failure and advanced atherosclerotic lesions. Arch Surg 1988; 123: 610-613.

[55] Acher CW, Belzer FO, Grist TM, et al. Late renal function in patients undergoing renal revascularization for control of hypertension and/or renal preservation. Cardiovasc Surg 1996; 4 (5): 602-606.

[56] Cormier F. Restorative aorto-iliac bypass surgery. Encycl Méd Chir: Techniques chirurgicales. Chirurgie vasculaire 43-035; 1998 :19 p.

[57] Kwaan JH, Connolly JE, Coutsoftides T. Concomitant revascularization of intestines during aorto-iliac reconstruction: deterrent to catastrophic bowel infarction. Can J Surg. 1980 Nov; 23(6): 534-6.

[58] Connolly JE, Price T. Aorto-iliac endarterectomy: alost art ?Ann Vasc Surg 2006; 20: 5662.

[59] Abid A, Denguir R, Kaouel K, Gharsallah N, Khanfir I, Chihaoui M, Kalfat T, Khayati A. Revascularisation of the lower limbs by extra-anatomical bypasses: A report on 80 cases. J Mal Vasc 2001; 26: 307-313.

[60] Benhamou AC, Mercier F, Kieffer E. Contribution of laparoscopic and video-assisted techniques to aorto-iliac surgery. J Mal Vasc 2001; 25: 212.

[61] Ariane J, Francis B. Anaesthesia and surgery of the abdominal aorta: anaesthetic specificities according to surgical specialists 2001; 7: 1-12.

[62] Berens ES, Herde JR. Laparoscopic vascular surgery: four case reports. J Vasc Surg 1995; 22:73-9.

[63] Dion YM, Gracia CR, Demalsy JC. Laparoscopic aortic surgery. J Vasc Surg 1996; 23: 539.

[64] Said S, Mall J, Peter F, Muller JM. Laparoscopic aorto-femoral bypass grafting: human cadaveric and initial clinical experiences. J Vasc Surg 1999; 29: 639-48.

[65] Coggia M, Javerliat I, Di Centa I et al. Total laparoscopic bypass for aorto-iliac occlusive disease: 93-case experience. J Vasc Surg 2004; 40: 899-906.

[66] Upchurch GR, Dimick JB, Wainess RM, et al. Diffusion of new technology in healthcare: the case of aorto-iliac occlusive disease. Surgery 2004; 136: 812-818.

[67] Kashyap VS, Pavkov ML, Bena JF, et al. The management of severe aorto-iliac occlusive disease: endovascular therapy rivals open reconstruction. J Vasc Surg 2008; 48: 1451-1457.

[68] Houston JG, MC Collum PT, Stonebridge PA, Raza Z, Shaw JW. Aortic bifurcation reconstruction: use of the Memothermself-expanding Nitinol stent for stenoses and occlusions. Cardiovasc Intervent Radiol 1999; 22: 89-95.

[69] Tegtmeyer CJ, Kellum CD, Kron IL, Mentzer RM, JR. Percutaneous transluminal angioplasty in the region of the aorticbifurcation. The two-balloon technique with results and long-term follow-up study. Radiology, 1985; 157: 661- 5.

[70] **Beckman JA**. Peripheral endovascular revascularization: some proof in the pudding? Circulation 2007; 115: 550-552.

[71] Spinosa DD, Leung DA, Harthun NL, et al. Simultaneous antegrade and retrograde access for subintimal recanalization of peripheral arterial occlusion. J Vasc Interv Radiol 2003; 14: 1449-1454.

[72] Bosch JL, Hunink MG. Meta-analysis of the results of PTA and stent placement for aorto iliac occlusive disease. Radiology 1997; 204: 87-96.

[73] Jacobs D, Motaganahalli RL, Cox DE, et al. True lumen reentry devices facilitate subintimal angioplasty and stenting of total chronic occlusions: initial report. J Vasc Surg 2006; 43: 1291-1296.

[74] Jongkind V, Akkersdijk GJ, Yeung KK, Wisselink W. A systematic review of endovascular treatment of extensive aorto-iliac occlusive disease. J Vasc Surg 2010; 52: 1376-83.

[75] The Task Force on the Diagnosis and Treatment of Peripheral Artery Diseases of the European Society of Cardiology (ESC). ESC Guidelines on the diagnosis and treatment of peripheral artery diseases. EurHeart Journal (2011) 32, 2851-2906.

[76] Tendera M, Aboyans V, Bartelink M, et al. ESC guidelines on the diagnosis and treatment of peripheral artery disease. Eur Heart J 2011; 32: 2851-906.

[77] Rooke TW, Hirsch AT, Misra S, et al. Management of patients with peripheral artery disease (compilation of 2005 and 2011 ACCF/AHA guideline recommendations): a report of the American College of Cardiology Foundation/American Heart Association Task Force on Practice Guidelines. J Am Coll Cardiol 2013;61:1555-70.

[78] Jeffrey W. Olin, Christopher J. White, Ehrin J. Armstrong, MSC, Daniella Kadian Dodov, William R. Hiatt. Peripheral Artery Disease. Evolving Role of

Exercise, Medical Therapy, and Endovascular Options. Journalof the American College of Cardiology VO L .67, NO. 11, 2016.

[79]De Donato G, Bosiers M, Setacci F, et al.24-Month data from the BRAVISSIMO: a large scale prospective registry on iliac stenting for TASC A & B and TASC C & D lesions. Ann Vasc Surg 2015; 29: 738-50.

[80] Inter-Society Consensus for the management of peripheral arterial disease (TASC II). J Vasc Surg 2007; 45(Suppl): 55A-567.

[81] Davidovic L, Vasic D, Maksimovic R, Kostic D, Markovic D, Markovic M. Aorto-bifemoral grafting: factors influencing long-term results. Vascular 2004; 12: 171-178.

[82] Liedenbaum MH, Verdam FJ, Spelt D et al. The outcome of the axillo-femoral bypass: a retrospective analysis of 45 patients. World J Surg 2009 33: 2490-2496.

[83] Martin D, Katz SG. Axillofemoral bypass for aorto-iliac occlusive disease. Am J Surg 2000; 180:100-103.

[84] Schneider JR, McDaniel MD, Walsh DB et al. Axillofemoral bypass: outcome and hemodynamic results in high-risk patients. J Vasc Surg 1992; 15: 952-962.

[85] Olson CJ, Edwards JM, Taylor LM et al. Repeat axillofemoral grafting as treatment for axillofemoral graft occlusion. Arch Surg 2002; 137: 1364-1367.

[86] Madenci AL, Ozaki CK, Gupta N, Raffetto JD, Belkin M, Mc Phee JT. Perioperative outcomes of elective inflow revascularization for lower extremity claudication in the American College of Surgeons National Surgical Quality Improvement Program database. Am J Surg. 2016 Sep; 212(3): 461-467.e2. doi: 10.1016/j.amjsurg.2015.10.016. Epub 2015 Dec 13.

[87] Anidjar S, Decaix B, Bertrand M, et al. Postoperative mortality and

morbidity in direct surgery for chronic aorto-iliac occlusive lesions. In: Kieffer E ed. Les Lésions Occlusives Aorto-iliaques Chroniques. Paris: AERCV, 1991. pp 181-189.

[88] Bredahl K, Jensen LP, Schroeder TV, Sillesen H, Nielsen H, Eiberg JP. Mortality and complications after aortic bifurcated bypass procedures for chronic aorto-iliac occlusive disease. J Vasc Surg 2015 Jul;62(1):75-82. doi: 10.1016/j.jvs.2015.02.025.

[89] Darling RC III, Kreienberg PB, Shah DM, Chang BB, Leather RP. Aortic reconstruction and concomitant renal artery revascularization using the retroperitoneal approach: techniques and results. Sem Vasc Surg 1996; 9 (3): 231-235.

[90] Chaikof EL, Smith RB, Salam AA, et al. Empirical reconstruction of the renal artery: long-term outcome. J Vasc Surg 1996; 24: 406-414.

[91] Calligaro, K.D, Azurin, D.J, Dougherty, M.J, Dandora, R, Bajgier, S.M, Simper, S et al. Pulmonary risk factors of elective abdominal aortic surgery. J Vasc Surg 1993; 18: 914- 920.

[92] David A Axelrod James C Stanley, Gilbert R Upchurch Jr, Shukri Khuri, Jennifer Daley, William Henderson, Sonia Demonner, Peter K Henke. Risk for stroke after elective non-carotid vascular surgery. Journal of Vascular Surgery Volume 39, Issue 1, January 2004, Pages 67-72.

[93] Cormier F, Fackas JC. Complications of aorto-iliac bypass surgery. Encycl Med Chir, Techniques chirurgicales, Chirurgie vasculaire 1999; 43-45: 22p.

[94] Cambria RP, Brewster DC, Abbott WM, Freehan M, Megerman J, La Muraglia G, et al. Trans-peritoneal versus retroperitoneal approach for aortic reconstruction: a randomized prospective study. J Vasc Surg 1990; 11: 314-25.

[95] Sicard GA, Reilly JM, Rubin BG, Thompson RW, Allen BT, Flye MW, et al. Trans-abdominal versus retroperitoneal incision for abdominal aortic surgery:

report of a prospective randomized trial. J Vasc Surg 1995; 21: 174-81.

[96] A. Nevelsteen, L. Woutersand R. Suy. Aortofemoral Dacron Reconstruction for Aortoiliac Occlusive Disease: A 25-year Survey. Eur J Vasc Surg 1991; 5, 179-186.

[97] D. Emerick Szilagyi, Joseph P. Elliott, Jr, Roger F. Smith, Daniel J. Reddy, and Michalene Mc Pharlin, R.N, Detroit, Mich. A thirty-year survey of the reconstructive surgical treatment of aorto-iliac occlusive disease. Journal of Vascular Surgery 428.

[98] W B Campbell, L J M T Tambeur, V R Geens. Local complications after arterial bypass grafting. Ann R Coll Surg Engl 1994; 76: 127-131

[99] Gelman S. The pathophysiology of aortic cross-clamping and unclamping. Anesthesiology 1995; 1026-50.

[100]Lacquet JP, Lacroix H, Nevelstenn A, Suy R. Inflammatory aortic aneurysm. A retrospective study of 100 cases. Acta Chir Belg 1997; 97: 286-92.

[101] De Palma RG, Levine SB, Feldman S. Preservation of erectile function after aorto-iliac reconstruction. Arch Surg 1978; 113: 958.

[102] Chiu KW, Davies RS, Nightingale PG, Bradbury AW, Adam DJ. Review of direct anatomical open surgical management of atherosclerotic aorto-iliac occlusive disease. Eur J Vasc Endovasc Surg 2010; 39: 460-471.

[103] Cormier F, Farkas JC. Complications of restorative aorto-iliac bypass surgery. EMC Techniques chirurgicales - Chirurgie vasculaire, 43-045.

[104] Nevelsteen A, Suy R. Graft occlusion following aorto-femoral Dacron bypass. Ann Vasc Surg 1991; 5: 32-37.

[105] Cron JP, Cron J, Blanchard D. Long-term results of aorto-bifemoral prostheses in surgery for atheromatous stenosis of the aortic arch. Arch Mal Cœur 1998; 91: 21-28.

[106] Nolan KD, Benjamin ME, Murphy TJ, et al. Femoro-femoral bypass for aorto-femoral graft limb occlusion: A ten-year experience. J Vasc Surg 1994; 19: 851.

[107] Enrique Criado, Blaire A Keagy, Chapel Hill. Aorto-iliac revascularisation by bypass from the descending thoracic aorta: indications and long-term results. Ann Chir Vasc 1994; 8: 38-47.

[108] Aguiar ET, Langer B, Lobato AC. Risk of false aneurysm and prosthetic infection after prosthetic aortofemoral bypass grafting: a retrospective study of 211 cases. J Mal Vasc 1996; 21: 36-39.

[109] Van Der Akker PJ, Van Schifgoarde R, Brande R. False aneurysm after prosthetic reconstruction for aorto-iliac obstructive disease. Ann Surg 1989; 210: 658-66.

[110] Thony F, Michoud M, Monnin V, Ferretti G, Rodière M. Imaging the pathological abdominal aorta. Feuillets de radiologie 2016; xxx:1-24.

[111] Seeger JM, Pretus HA. Welborn MB et al. Long term outcome after treatment of aortic graft infection with staged extra-anatomic bypass grafting and aortic graft removal. J Vasc Surg 2000; 32: 451-461.

[112] Kieffer E, Gomes D. Chiche L et al. Allograft replacement for infra-renal aortic graft infection: early and lateresultsin179 patients. J Vasc Surg 2004; 39: 1009-1017.

[113] Constans J. Secondary aorto duodenal fistulas: report of 7 cases. Rev Med Interne 1999; 20: 121-7.

[114] Bergqvist D, Bjorkman H, Bolin T, Dalman P, Elfstrom J, Forsberg O, et al. Secondary aorto enteric fistulae-changes from 1973to 1993. Eur J Vasc Endovasc Surg 1996; 11: 425-8.

[115] Tacchini S. CT findings of secondary aorto-enteric fistulae. Radiol Med 2005; 110:492- 500.

[116] Kuestner LM, Reilly LM, Jicha DL, Ehrenfeld WK, Goldstone J, Stoney RS. Secondary aorto-enteric fistula: contemporaneous outcome with use of extra- anatomic bypass and infected graft excision. J VascSurg 1995; 21: 184-96.

# TABLE OF CONTENTS


I-INTRODUCTION ................................................................... 2

II-EPIDEMIOLOGY .............................................................. 3

III-CLINICAL STUDY ........................................................... 7

IV-ADDITIONAL TESTS ...................................................... 10

V-TREATMENT................................................................... 15

VI-RESULTS OF SURGICAL TREATMENT ....................... 29

VII-CONCLUSION ............................................................... 40

BIBLIOGRAPHY ................................................................. 42

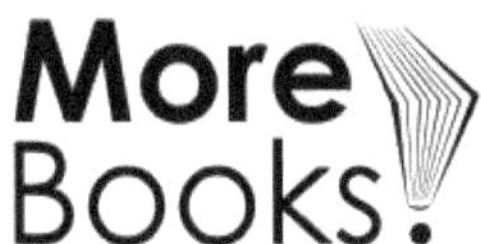

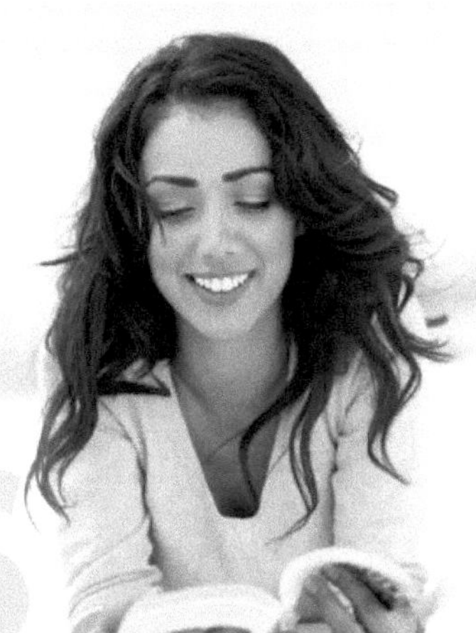

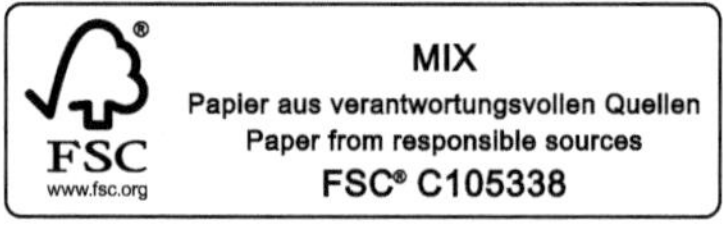


Printed by Books on Demand GmbH, Norderstedt / Germany